Contents

GUIDED MEDITATION

FOR

WEIGHT LOSS

Positive, Natural Weight Loss,

Calm the Mind Using Meditative

Subliminal Affirmations & Relaxing Music

to Help you Stay Fit and Thin for Life

Disclaimer:

Results may vary and are not guaranteed. You agree to use these meditations of your own free will and choice. This content is not intended in any way as a substitute for professional medical advice, diagnosis, or treatment. Always seek the advice of your physician or other qualified health care provider with any questions you may have regarding your current health condition, and before starting any new health care regimen.

INTRODUCTION

"Whatever we plant in our subconscious mind and nourish with repetition and emotion will one day become a reality."

- Earl Nightingale

Are you ready to see yourself in a whole new way?

There are many factors present when it comes to being overweight. The world we live in, filled with artificial foods, not to mention the stress level of most people, are obvious culprits. Because of our lifestyle, we often indulge in unhealthy behaviors, such as stress eating, eating for comfort, or binge-watching our favorite television shows. All this plays a part in unhealthy living. The weight loss industry has made billions on the claim that you just need to change your eating habits to change your body. This couldn't be further from the truth. While the belief of calories in, calories out, plays a role in overall body shape, it is a far cry from being the end-all, be-all of weight management. Your body is energetic. The study of Quantum Physics tells us that everything is made up of energy, from the tiniest particle to our houses, cars, clothes, food, and yes, our bodies.

What role does energy play in the process of losing weight? If your energetic frequency is set at "fat" mode, (you subconsciously see yourself as fat), no dieting, exercising or deprivation is going to get you thin. And even if dieting gets some of the pounds off, it's highly likely you will put them back on without properly addressing your inner needs. All emotions play a role in where you are today. The emotions from your childhood make up a large portion of your current habits. If there are any traumas, unforgiveness, or any other of the plethora of human emotions present, your current thought process could be keeping you from getting thin. Because the body acts to protect itself and is designed to make sure it has what it needs to survive, it creates habits to sustain that safety. However, it is only because of past conditioning that the mind and body work together to create this illusion of safety. That past conditioning can be changed, and that is where meditation comes in.

Why Meditation Works

Meditation is a mind/body practice that has been used for thousands of years to help promote calmness and an overall sense of well-being. It traditionally requires you to relax while listening to soothing words, music, or both, with the intention of creating new ideas in the brain.

All change starts in the mind and these meditations are designed to help the mind start the process of change towards a healthier you. Because the act of meditating accesses the subconscious mind (the area of the brain responsible for automatic bodily functions such as breathing and heart rate), rather than the conscious, it gets to the heart of the issues, habits, and areas of your past that you may not be willing to let go of. At least, not consciously.

Your mind is an incredible machine. It creates what it believes to be the best for you. But in order for you to be at your best, you have to feed it the right frequencies. Old, stuck emotions such as anger, grief or frustration can create a loop of thoughts that keep you trapped in a low frequency. These meditations work to bring you out of these stuck patterns to an awareness of your power and magnificence.

Furthermore, these meditations, when used with healthy lifestyle choices, are designed to help you create a new pattern of thought and action. Using visualization practices, you will start to think and "act" like a thin person. You will no longer "see" yourself as someone who has a weight problem. Because of this, you will naturally and easily lean toward healthier food choices (without feeling deprived!) Your relationship with your body image, food, and exercise will begin to improve, and you'll feel more motivated to work toward solutions.

Other benefits, such as a change in unhealthy habits, awareness about cravings, and improved mental focus are common when applying a meditation regimen. These new habits will support the evolving you, and you'll work toward creating the best version of yourself! The soothing words will take you on a journey of self-discovery, helping you realize where you may need improvement.

The tracks are designed to be listened to in sequence. It is recommended you listen to each one, starting with Meditation #1: The Beginning of Body Awareness, once a day for at least one week, before moving on to the next. Your body may want to go at a slower pace, so make sure to "tune in" to how you are feeling and go with what feels natural and good to you. Each track builds on the one before it and helps mold your mind into a machine that will work for you, day in and day out.

Get ready for a change in your thinking… and your body!

Meditation #1: The Beginning of Body Awareness

Find a comfortable seated position that makes you feel relaxed and able to focus on your breath…

Dim the lights and put away all distractions for the next few minutes… this time is for you… to give yourself what you need… to help you tune in to who you are…

Take your time to find the right position and tune into this important present moment….

Take a deep breath in… and now blow it out… again, a deep breath in, you are getting more relaxed… and out…

Today we are going to understand more about body image and weight… how you see yourself… and where you ultimately want to be…

Weight is not all about calories… the body is intelligent… it knows how to keep us safe… secure… our emotions play a significant roll…

Sometimes our emotions and energy can prevent us from following a healthy lifestyle… because of the past… because of what we've been through…

Now is the time to allow your body to let go of these obstacles… and embark on a journey of discovery… relaxation… and openness to embrace change within your soul… and your body…

We often find ourselves struggling and stuck with a sense of discomfort… of uneasiness… of disharmony… of not feeling good enough…

You can shift this energy…

Focus on the emotions that fill your life… what are you feeling about yourself?... focus on those emotions that won't allow you to be truly present in the moment…

Visualize a storm inside you… it's intimidating… it feels heavy… the black clouds are rolling in… and for a time there is no sign of sunshine…

It's raining heavily… it's windy… it's dark… there is thunder and lightning all around… the tumultuous weather has you feeling uncertain…

You feel shaky… you feel confused… you are afraid…

Your emotions are all over the place… but then… out of the darkness… you start realizing you can do this… you can face the storm… How?...

Because you have the power to make it stop… you have the energy to do so…

You just need to believe in yourself… in your ability to let the storm pass… and leave space for a balanced, harmonious place within your heart…

Take a long deep breath in through the nose… and exhale out your mouth with a long sigh…

Breathe in… feel how the air is now filling your body…

And see with your exhale the storm inside you calming down….

You can spot a few sunrays peeking through the heavy clouds… the light is beginning to come forth…

You know you can do this… you breathe into this scenario again to cleanse this space and create harmony and balance within…

Again, take a long deep breath in through the nose… and exhale out your mouth….

The rain is quieting… and soon you can't hear the sound of raindrops anymore…

A quiet peace comes into the scene… as the storm clears…

There is no time and space for discomfort here…

You take another deep breath in… and as you breathe out, visualize your breath clearing the clouds…

There is no wind anymore…

You can feel a sense of peace moving toward you….

Now, collect all the parts of this storm… the darkness… the rain… the wind… the thunder… and lighting… gather these elements together into one big energy ball as you breathe deeply in… and as you exhale… release the darkness… the sense of discomfort… confusion… disharmony… and unease…

Now, the storm has passed… and in its place… a sweet calm… the sun is shining… you can sense the bright light and clear sky generating a sense of harmony and balance within…

You made this place… you were able to do this… you were able to go here…

The same is true of how you view yourself…

Where you are right now may not be where you want to be…

It may look scary to you… or seem dark… with no way out…

No matter how uncertain a storm may look… you have the power to overcome it…

Begin now to understand how your body has served you… through the storms…

It may feel like you are in the middle of a dark and turbulent time… but you can bring yourself back… back to where it feels peaceful again…

You can see yourself where you want to be… you can visualize the person you truly are… you can see a powerful, thin, strong body… you can bring yourself to this place in your mind… and the more you do… the faster your outer reality will move to match your inner reality…

You will come to appreciate and realize the magnificence of your body…

This is the first step…

To remember how powerful you are…

To remember that you can create the body you want…

It begins in the mind…

It starts with your thoughts…

Thoughts that can serve you and bring you what you want…

Start by overcoming the storm inside you… begin to question how you see yourself… question the darkness… question the chaos… why does it get to live in your body?

Can you begin to allow the light? Yes… you have that power…

What body do you want? Let the question permeate your being… begin to see what you really want… allow the image to come to your mind… dwell there… in peace…

And whenever the storm begins to come… bring yourself back to this peaceful place… where you are living your perfect life… in your perfect body…

Surrender yourself to the idea of being right where you want to be…

Now, come to an awareness of your body…

Take a deep breath in, and blow it out slowly… continue bringing your awareness back to the present moment…

Wiggle your fingers… and now your toes…

Open your eyes… feeling refreshed and ready to move toward your goal…

Meditation #2: Letting Go of the Past to Achieve Your Dream Body

Find a comfortable seated position of your choice… choose a position that makes you feel relaxed…at ease…keep your shoulders relaxed… chest open… rest your arms at your side or on your lap… take a deep breath in through the nose… and out through the mouth… let's begin…

Take these moments as precious time to let go of the past… to construct new thoughts… a chance to achieve an ideal body weight and shape…

Again, take a long deep breath in through the nose… and out through your mouth… let your breath continue until there is no air left in your lungs… then breathe in and on the exhale, let go… becoming fully relaxed as these words wash over you…

Begin to notice how you feel… how you are tuning in to the power of your breath… feel how you are now present… committed to this moment… committed to making a change…

You are beginning the process of living your best life… by letting go of your past… and listening to your inner voice… you acknowledge that once the past is gone… you are ready to allow the new you…

The past gives us no self-respect… it creeps up on us at any moment… it creates a distorted vision of ourselves… maybe we are doubting a choice we made… seeing things that didn't work out… there is doubt… fear… regret…

But deep down you are starting to develop a new understanding… one that teaches you more… that because of your experience… you are the person you are today… one that doesn't have to be weighed down…

That weight has kept you stuck… in past events… you are carrying a heavy load… one that you can let go of… and let drop… so you are finally free…

Focus on a situation or person from your past… find the sensation of how it feels… of not trusting yourself… not trusting your intuition…

See the heavy chains holding you to this situation… don't force yourself to change what happened… it is what it is… and it is okay to feel what you feel… there is nothing wrong in having these emotions… in having these blockages…

They have served their purpose… and now… instead of continuing to carry these chains… these emotions… these feelings… it's time to transform them… so you can let go of the heaviness…

A vast body of water is coming into your view… it is calm and clear… it feels expansive… hopeful… it is ready to serve you…

Walk to the water's edge… and allow your emotions… your feelings… and the chains… to flow into this water…

You see the chains falling off… you feel relief as they fall… the water envelops them… and changes the heaviness…

Now you feel lighter… like a load has been dropped… not because the past has changed… but because you have changed…

You made that choice… you just did that… you dropped your chains…

You don't need protection from those chains anymore… you don't need to carry that load… you are safe now…

It is safe to achieve your ideal body… it is safe to visualize what you want… it is safe to believe in your dreams… the past can't hurt you anymore…

Take a deep breath in… and as you blow it out… release any blockages you are sensing… just allow them to go… see your body developing new pathways of light… see the light moving throughout your entire body… healing as it goes…

The light is continuing to increase… filling you with peace… your happiness is its goal…

You've got this… you can create the life you want… you can be who you want to be… it's finally time…

No more chains from your past… you have safely let them go… and it is safe to start the process of allowing the weight to come off… of allowing the perfect you…

See your body… standing in peace and tranquility… see the unburdening of your body… see yourself feeling light… carefree… ready for the next chapter…

See yourself as hopeful… excited… for a new door has opened… and all you have to do is walk through it… it is safe on the other side…

Take a deep breath in through the nose… and out through the mouth… allowing any other unwanted sensations to leave your presence…

The past no longer has control over you…

It is safe to be thin and to have what you want….

Say these words out loud…

THE PAST HAS NO CONTROL OVER ME…

Take a deep breath in… and out… say aloud…

I RELEASE THE CHAINS I'VE BEEN CARRYING…

Another breath in… and out… say aloud…

I TRUST MY VISION…

Feel a sense of freedom and relaxation taking over… the light is continuing to grow… filling your body and the room…

You are ready to honor yourself… to honor your vision… to allow the best version of yourself…

See yourself embarking on a new journey… see yourself releasing weight… feel yourself gaining confidence while losing weight…

See your end goal… see yourself how you want to be… become that person in your mind… who is that person?…

What qualities does this person have?... How does this person behave?...

Rather than being a product of your past... it's time to be a product of your future... the future that you create... you have the control... and power... to live the life you want... to be the person you want to be...

It's all up to you... and yes... you can do it...

Bring your awareness to the room you are in... begin to feel the sensations coming back... wiggle your fingers... now wiggle your toes... feel your body coming back to the present moment...

Now, open your eyes and become aware of the room you are in... feeling refreshed, motivated, and ready to accomplish your goals...

Meditation #3: Visualizing Your Perfect Body

A weight loss journey can be challenging… for both your body and your soul… you may at times lose your center… your attention… your motivation…

This guided meditation is for you… it's your gentle reminder… that you've got this… you can create what you want… you can make it happen…

It's time to be your own number one supporter… on this journey… that takes one step at a time… one pound at a time… with no judgment… and an open heart…

Find yourself a comfortable position where you are either reclining back, or lying down… remove all distractions… this is your time… a time when you can move toward your goals…

Take a deep breath in through your nose, and exhale out through your mouth… feel your body begin to relax… again, a deep breath in… and now out… good…

It's time to explore your higher self… the one that is already what and where you want to be… open your heart and focus on how you really feel… take another long breath in… and long breath out…

Let's begin by visualizing yourself in your new body…

See yourself in front of a mirror… you are looking at your magnificent body… you are in the best shape of your life…

your body is thinner…. it's lean… fit… strong… beautiful…

See yourself getting ready to go somewhere… you are putting on your best clothes… they easily glide over your toned body… there is no tightness… you feel light… and assured…

You feel confidence taking over… you can accomplish anything… you are about to have an amazing day…

With this new shape… you can have it all… be what you have always dreamed of being…

You smile at yourself… you are proud of how far you've come… it hasn't always been easy… you've been through a lot… there have been challenges…

But you are beginning to see… that those challenges made the person you are… and they are just fueling your desire… to be the best you can be…

You walk out to a street… and begin strolling… enjoying the bustle of life…

You notice people are looking at you… smiling… their heads turning to see how stunning you are… not only on the outside… but they can see your happiness… and that makes you even more attractive…

You stop walking and a powerful image comes into your mind… the image is of you… the person that these people see… only you see yourself the same way… you value who you are… you accept who you are… the image continues in intensity and power… until you feel it might burst forth from within you…

You feel empowered… you feel self-assured…

And then the emotion of love comes into play… you feel unconditional, unwavering love for this person… who is on this journey… and who has overcome so much…

You are the best version of yourself…

This vision can manifest in real life… for whatever is conceived in the mind… can be achieved in reality…

Whenever you are feeling down on yourself… and life seems challenging… conjure again this image of yourself… feel the emotions you felt when you saw yourself as your best version… feel how your clothes felt… see how confident you were… how good you felt about yourself…

Take a deep breath in through your nose…. exhale out the mouth and say aloud…

I AM BEAUTIFUL…

Listen to the sound of your voice… to your commitment coming to life…

Take a deep breath in through your nose…. exhale out the mouth and say aloud…

I AM THE FIT, THIN VERSION OF MYSELF…

Feel the power of your words… their vibration in your chest… the clarity taking over all though your body…

One more time… take a deep breath in through your nose…. exhale out the mouth and say aloud…

I CREATE THE BEST VERSION OF MYSELF IN THIS MOMENT…

Accept your own command… each time you say this statement… see yourself where you want to be… your words are powerful… use them to your advantage…

As you take your next breath, inhale peace… on the exhale, release any negativity you may feel about yourself… and just be an observer to any limiting beliefs… they are only telling you a story… and you are the author of your story… you get to choose how the story goes…

Let your expectations rise to support your vision… let them inspire you to believe in yourself… in your weight loss journey….

You now realize you can get what you want… you have the ability to do it… you have the power to do it…

We are going to state a few more affirmations…

Take a deep breath in through your nose…. exhale out the mouth and say aloud…

I AM STRONG…

Feel the power in your words… deep breath in… and out… say aloud…

I CAN DO THIS…

Believe yourself… deep breath in… and out… say aloud…

I EMBRACE THE BEST VERSION OF MYSELF…

Now, see yourself there… and feel the acceptance… for it is you who must accept the person you are… for it to become a reality…

Feel how your body and soul are in tune with one another… you've done some great work… continue to feel the changes you've made… support them by bringing yourself back to your vision… of your highest and best self…

Slowly begin to bring your awareness back into your body… start to feel the chair you're sitting on… and become aware of the room you're sitting in… now wiggle your fingers… and your toes…

Open your eyes… feeling powerfully refreshed… you are ready to tackle life as the new, best version of yourself…

Meditation #4: Choosing New Habits to Support Weight Loss

Find a seated position you like…recline back or lie down… make sure there are no distractions… and close your eyes…

Take a deep breath in through your nose…. and out through your mouth… begin to relax all your muscles… this is your time… time to tune into what you need… to help you on your weight loss journey…

Your mind is truly powerful… and helps you become successful… when you give it the right tools… when you allow the right habits to form…

Sometimes we make choices that inhibit our progress… it seems hard to move past a certain point… so we sabotage our efforts… we act impulsively… we make our life harder… and then we give up control… of being who we want to be… because our efforts seem futile…

This is the time to make adjustments… it's time to act intentionally… to make your dreams… plans… and goals… a reality…

See yourself standing on a road… you are looking ahead… you see a fork, with one road leading right… and one road leading left… the road on your left is the road you've been traveling on… you know its twists and turns… you know its roadblocks… and even though there are pitfalls… it seems safer… than venturing to the right… into the unknown…

But the road you've been traveling on isn't serving you anymore…it's leading you down paths you don't agree with… that the highest version of yourself doesn't resonate with…

So, you must make a choice… to take the road that is familiar… or have courage… and take the road less traveled…

Along the road less traveled… there are still obstacles… there are still pitfalls… but you can overcome them… you know how to navigate them… because of your experience… because you are strong…

And along the road less traveled… there is greater success… because when you make a different decision… you break free of your fear… and move past what was stopping you…

You decide to take the road to the right… the road you haven't traveled before… you're not sure what to expect… but you are now committed… you know there may be challenges… but you are willing to face them…

When we are faced with change… change that will transform us… it's always easier to stay on the familiar path… to stay close to what's known… but you'll never know where the road can lead… what happiness you can achieve… if you are too afraid to change your course…

You are choosing a new path… you are choosing new habits… ones that may seem uncertain… but you know there will be a payoff… you know it will be worth it…

Facing your past… making different choices… that are good for you… raises the frequency of your body… and changes the very fiber of your being…

Eating different foods… and making the choice to get off the couch… may not seem like big things… but choosing them will change your attitude… and attitude is everything…

Take a deep breath in… and blow it out…

The road is getting easier now… you are moving down it at an even pace… the obstacles don't seem so huge… because now you know what to expect…

You find it easy to choose the "light" foods… ones that are filled with high frequency and amazing nutrition… your body craves them… you are drawn to them…

Your mind is beckoning to take a walk along the seashore… or down the lane… there is so much to see in this big, beautiful world… you want to get out and explore… and doing so fills your lungs with oxygen… and your heart with joy… it feels so good…

When you bump into an obstacle on your path… when the familiar knocks at your mind's door… you simply don't answer… it isn't welcome anymore… instead… you feed your mind nourishing thoughts… thoughts of encouragement… thoughts of being on the right path…

Your energy is rising… your power is increasing… little by little… you are making the right choices for you…

All to support you on your weight loss journey… all to help you achieve your perfect body weight and size… all to help you accept yourself… your magnificent self…

Take a deep breath in through the nose… and smile as you exhale out through your mouth with a liberating sigh…

Take a deep breath in… and now out…

Say out loud…

ALL CRAVINGS FOR UNHEALTHY BEHAVIORS ARE GONE…

Take a deep breath in… and out…

Say out loud…

I CAN AND DO MAKE HEALTHY CHOICES…

Take another deep breath in… and out…

Say out loud…

I AM ON THE RIGHT PATH…

You have control over any cravings… you see food differently… you choose healthy options… both in mind… and body…

You see these choices as an opportunity… a chance to take your life back… to create what you truly want…

Inhale deeply… and exhale completely…

See yourself standing on the right path… you are a healthy, thin person… who has made good choices…

You feel a sense of satisfaction… of conquering your fears… of overcoming the unknown… a sense of contentment… for embracing who you truly are… and finally becoming the best version of yourself…

Smile at this vision … you already are that person… you live in that body… your mind sees you as that person… now it's time to let reality catch up…

Take a deep breath in… and long breath out…

Begin to be aware of the room you're sitting in… and feel your body start to wake up… you can feel your hands and fingers… now your legs, feet and toes… bring your awareness fully to the present moment… and open your eyes… you are refreshed, ready to create the life of your dreams.

Meditation #5: Embracing the New You – Empowerment Meditation

Find a place where you can be alone and remove all distractions… take a seat in a comfortable position of your choice… take a deep breath in through your nose… and blow it out through your mouth… allow this time of transformation… to help you move in your desired direction… feel your body relaxing… now, close your eyes…

This moment is all yours… a moment to accept the new version of yourself… and allow your happiness… your new life is yours for the taking…

Inhale deeply through the nose… and exhale out through the mouth…

You've made an investment… of time… energy… practices… that have paid off…

You've planted a seed … that you have watered… and cared for… and because of your effort… the new plant has sprung forth… because of the law of nature… and of growth… and now… you are enjoying the fruits of your labor…

Now you get to embrace who you are… to welcome your new life…

It's all you wanted… it's all you hoped for…

You are thin… healthy… beautiful… happy… you are in the best shape of your life…

But this change is not only exterior… it's not only the way you look…

It's the way you feel… it's how you've changed on the inside…

You are different…

You feel stronger… you feel empowered… you feel amazing…

Positive energy is all around you… and you pull from it to move through your day…

You know you did it… you were able to create a different life…

The one you used to live… seems so far away now… you can hardly remember… the person you once were…

Because now your energy… is completely transformed… it supports the new you… and you've made the transition… into your new world…

Your weight loss journey was about more than becoming thin… it was a journey that made you appreciate yourself… and helped you rediscover your unique qualities… it showed you how to give yourself the love… gratitude… and respect… you've deserved all along…

The journey made you learn… about what makes you powerful… you were able to defeat the obstacles… you were able to overcome the setbacks… and the limiting beliefs…

You had challenges… you had to work through things… the way you felt… your emotions… you had to face things head on… and not let them weigh you down anymore…

Our reality is full of obstacles… and moments of negativity… but these are hidden blessings… because they teach us how to overcome… build our strength… and achieve more…

You now know… you can change the way you face them… you have the tools… to continue on your path… and accept the good… that inevitably comes with conquering any obstacle…

Inhale deeply through the nose... and now exhale out through the mouth...

You are an observer of your reality… you are watching your story… become the watcher… and when something negative shows up… breathe into it… the seed of hope… faith… and love…

Now, all this is a part of you… you can call on your strong, higher self… at any time…

You can continue on this journey… because you are not done… there are many wonderful things awaiting you… that long to be part of your story…

But for this moment… bask in the joy of accomplishment… and feel how good it feels… to be successful… to be the person… you want to be…

Inhale deeply through the nose… now exhale through the mouth…

Focus on what has made this journey special… what did you learn about yourself?… how do you view yourself?… what do you say about yourself now?… give yourself the credit…

You are ready to acknowledge it… to acknowledge your power… if you can do this… you can do anything… you can have all that you want…

You have become aware of how to make changes… and now you know the formula… to begin with the image in your mind… of your end goal…

Plant it… water it… nurture it… give it the care it needs… so it can grow… and spring forth with abundant goodness… to manifest your desires…

And know… that no matter where you go… or what you do… you will always have the power… to change your situation… because you have this wonderful tool… the tool of your mind… all can change in an instant… the moment you decide to change it in thought… because when you decide on an outcome… and you see that outcome… and live for that outcome… nothing can stop you…

The part of you who is beyond the flesh… that special part of you… who knows no limits… is your partner… and friend… and wants you to become unstoppable…

You are unstoppable…

And it feels incredible…

Now, begin to sense yourself in your room… you are slowly coming back to awareness of your surroundings… you begin to feel your arms… hands and fingers… now your legs…

your feet… your toes… wiggle them and feel the amazingness of your body… you are completely powerful… and your power has no limits… you are now fully aware… you feel completely rejuvenated… refreshed… ready to take on any goal you choose.

Thank You!

Thank you for using these meditation tracks to help you on your weight loss journey. I hope you've enjoyed the process and learned a lot about yourself. Remember, you always have the power to create the life you want… keep creating!

Namaste

May I ask for your review?

If you enjoyed these meditations, would you please take a moment to leave a review? They help me know what my readers like about my work, and how I can improve. Just enter this URL in your browser to leave your review. Thank you!

https://amzn.to/30gFPn2